DR. BARBARA'S SIMPLE 3 DAYS JUICE DETOX

The easy guide to harnessing the power of healing juice and smoothies to detox and cleanse your whole body, skin, kidney, liver, lungs for optimal well-being

Mauricio Andrea

Table of Contents

COPYRIGHT © 2023

All rights reserved. No part of this publication may be reproduced, distributed, or transmitted in any form or by any means, including photocopying, recording, or other electronic or mechanical methods, without the prior written permission of the publisher, except in the case of brief quotations embodied in critical reviews and certain other noncommercial uses permitted by copyright law.

CHAPTER ONE

Introduction to Juice Detox: Understanding Its Benefits and Purpose

Juice detox, also known as juice cleansing or juice fasting, has gained significant popularity in recent years as a method for detoxifying the body and promoting overall health and wellness. This practice involves consuming only freshly squeezed juices from fruits and vegetables for a certain period, typically ranging from a few days to several weeks. While juice detox has been met with both enthusiasm and skepticism, understanding its benefits and purpose is crucial for anyone considering embarking on such a regimen.

Understanding Juice Detox

Juice detox is rooted in the concept of detoxification, which is the process of eliminating toxins and impurities from the body. Proponents of juice detox believe that by consuming only nutrient-rich juices, the body can rid itself of accumulated toxins, promote healing, and rejuvenate vital organs such as the liver and kidneys. This process is thought to support overall health and well-being, as well as aid in weight loss and improve digestion.

The Benefits of Juice Detox

Advocates of juice detox cite numerous potential benefits associated with this practice. Firstly, consuming fresh juices provides the body with a concentrated source of essential vitamins, minerals, and antioxidants, which are crucial for maintaining optimal health. Fruits and vegetables are rich in nutrients such as vitamin C, vitamin A, potassium, and folate, all of which play vital roles in various bodily functions, including immune function, energy production, and cell repair.

Moreover, juice detox is believed to give the digestive system a much-needed break from processing solid foods, allowing it to rest and repair. This can lead to improved digestion, reduced bloating, and increased nutrient absorption. Additionally, proponents suggest that juice detox can help reset unhealthy eating patterns, reduce cravings for processed foods, and promote a greater appreciation for whole, natural foods.

Furthermore, some individuals report experiencing increased energy levels, mental clarity, and improved mood during and after a juice detox. This may be attributed to the elimination of toxins from the body, as well as the influx of nutrients from fresh juices. Some proponents also claim that juice detox can support weight loss by reducing calorie intake, eliminating cravings, and promoting fat loss.

The Purpose of Juice Detox

The primary purpose of juice detox is to support the body's natural detoxification processes and promote overall health and well-being. By consuming nutrient-rich juices while abstaining from solid foods, individuals aim to cleanse their bodies of toxins, boost their immune systems, and rejuvenate vital organs. Juice detox is often viewed as a holistic approach to health that addresses not only physical but also mental and emotional well-being.

Additionally, juice detox is sometimes used as a short-term intervention to kickstart healthier habits and break through plateaus in weight loss or fitness goals. Many people turn to juice detox as a way to reset their bodies after periods of indulgence or to counteract the effects of a poor diet and lifestyle choices. While the primary focus is on detoxification, juice fasting can also serve as a catalyst for long-term lifestyle changes, such as adopting a more plant-based diet or reducing reliance on processed foods.

Overall, the purpose of juice detox is to promote detoxification, rejuvenation, and overall health and wellness. While the specific goals may vary from individual to individual, the underlying principle remains the same: to support the body's innate ability to heal and thrive.

Conclusion

In conclusion, juice detox is a practice that involves consuming only freshly squeezed juices from fruits and vegetables for a certain period with the aim of detoxifying the body and promoting overall health and wellness. Proponents of juice detox believe that this practice can provide numerous benefits, including increased nutrient intake, improved digestion, increased energy levels, and mental clarity. The primary purpose of juice detox is to support the body's natural detoxification processes and promote overall health and well-being. While juice detox may not be suitable for everyone, understanding its benefits and purpose can help individuals make informed decisions about whether it is the right choice for them.

CHAPTER TWO

Meet Dr. Barbara: Her Background and Expertise in Herbal Medicine

Dr. Barbara is a distinguished expert in the field of herbal medicine, with a rich background and extensive experience in utilizing botanical remedies to promote health and well-being. Her journey into the world of herbal medicine began with a deep-rooted passion for plants and their healing properties, coupled with a commitment to holistic healthcare practices.

Background of Dr. Barbara

Dr. Barbara's interest in herbal medicine can be traced back to her upbringing in a family that placed a strong emphasis on natural remedies and traditional healing practices. From a young age, she was exposed to the medicinal properties of various herbs and plants, learning firsthand from her grandparents who cultivated a diverse garden of healing herbs.

Driven by a desire to deepen her understanding of herbal medicine, Dr. Barbara pursued formal education in the field, earning advanced degrees in botany, pharmacology, and traditional medicine. Her academic journey provided her with a solid foundation in the scientific principles underlying herbal remedies, as well as a comprehensive understanding of the therapeutic potential of plant-based medicines.

Expertise in Herbal Medicine

Dr. Barbara's expertise in herbal medicine spans a wide range of areas, including botanical identification, phytochemistry, pharmacology, and clinical applications of herbal remedies. She has dedicated her career to researching the medicinal properties of various plants and herbs, with a focus on identifying novel compounds and understanding their mechanisms of action.

One of Dr. Barbara's key areas of expertise lies in herbal pharmacology, where she applies her knowledge of plant constituents and their pharmacological effects to develop evidence-based herbal formulations. Her research has contributed to the growing body of scientific literature on herbal medicine, helping to bridge the gap between traditional knowledge and modern healthcare practices.

In addition to her research endeavors, Dr. Barbara is also an experienced clinician who has worked with patients seeking alternative and complementary treatments for a wide range of health conditions. She employs a holistic approach to patient care, taking into account not only the physical symptoms but also the underlying imbalances that contribute to disease.

Dr. Barbara's expertise extends beyond the laboratory and clinic, as she is also a passionate educator and advocate for herbal medicine. She regularly conducts workshops, seminars, and public lectures to share her knowledge and empower individuals to take control of their health through natural means. Her dedication to education extends to mentoring aspiring herbalists and healthcare professionals, guiding them on their own journeys into the world of herbal medicine.

Conclusion

In conclusion, Dr. Barbara is a renowned expert in the field of herbal medicine, with a wealth of knowledge and experience in harnessing the healing power of plants. Her background in botany, pharmacology, and traditional medicine, coupled with her clinical expertise and passion for education, make her a trusted authority in the field. Through her research, clinical practice, and advocacy efforts, Dr. Barbara continues to make significant contributions to the advancement of herbal medicine and the promotion of holistic healthcare practices.

CHAPTER THREE

The Science of Juice Detox: How It Supports Cleansing and Health

Juice detox, also known as juice cleansing or juice fasting, is often touted for its potential to support cleansing and promote overall health and well-being. While some view juice detox as a trendy fad, there is scientific evidence to suggest that it can indeed offer certain benefits when done correctly and for the right reasons. Understanding the science behind juice detox can provide insight into how it supports cleansing and contributes to health.

Nutrient Density of Fresh Juices

One of the primary reasons juice detox is believed to support cleansing and health is the nutrient density of fresh juices. Fruits and vegetables are rich sources of vitamins, minerals, antioxidants, and phytonutrients, all of which play essential roles in various bodily functions. By consuming freshly squeezed juices, individuals can flood their bodies with these nutrients, supporting overall health and well-being.

For example, fruits like oranges, grapefruits, and lemons are high in vitamin C, which is essential for immune function and collagen production. Leafy greens like kale, spinach, and Swiss chard are packed with vitamins A, K, and folate, as well as minerals like potassium and magnesium, which are crucial for heart health and muscle function. Additionally, phytonutrients found in fruits and vegetables have antioxidant and anti-inflammatory properties, helping to protect cells from damage and reduce the risk of chronic diseases.

Digestive Rest and Healing

Another aspect of juice detox is the concept of giving the digestive system a break from processing solid foods. Solid foods require energy and resources for digestion, absorption, and elimination, whereas liquids like fresh juices are easier for the body to digest and assimilate. By consuming only juices for a period, individuals allow their digestive systems to rest and redirect energy towards other essential functions, such as cellular repair and detoxification.

During juice detox, the digestive system undergoes a process known as autophagy, wherein old and damaged cells are broken down and recycled. This cellular cleansing and renewal process can contribute to improved overall health and vitality. Additionally, the restorative effects of juice detox on the digestive system can lead to improvements in gut health, reduced inflammation, and enhanced nutrient absorption.

Hydration and Detoxification

Hydration is another critical aspect of juice detox that supports cleansing and health. Many fruits and vegetables have high water content, which helps to hydrate the body and flush out toxins through urine and sweat. Proper hydration is essential for maintaining the balance of bodily fluids, regulating body temperature, and supporting various biochemical processes.

Furthermore, certain fruits and vegetables used in juice detox, such as cucumbers, celery, and watermelon, have diuretic properties, meaning they promote urine production and help to eliminate excess water and toxins from the body. This diuretic effect can aid in the detoxification process by supporting the function of the kidneys and reducing fluid retention.

Conclusion

In conclusion, the science behind juice detox reveals how it supports cleansing and contributes to overall health and well-being. The nutrient density of fresh juices provides essential vitamins, minerals, antioxidants, and phytonutrients that support various bodily functions and protect against chronic diseases. Giving the digestive system a rest allows for cellular repair and detoxification, leading to improvements in gut health and overall vitality. Additionally, hydration plays a crucial role in detoxification by flushing out toxins and supporting the function of the kidneys. While juice detox may not be suitable for everyone, understanding its scientific principles can help individuals make informed decisions about incorporating it into their wellness routines.

CHAPTER FOUR

Getting Started: Preparing Mentally and Physically for the Detox

Embarking on a juice detox requires careful preparation, both mentally and physically, to ensure a successful and fulfilling experience. Preparation is key to setting realistic expectations, addressing potential challenges, and maximizing the benefits of the detox process. Whether you're new to juice detox or a seasoned practitioner, taking the time to prepare yourself adequately can make all the difference in your journey towards improved health and well-being.

Mental Preparation

1. **Set Clear Intentions:** Before starting a juice detox, it's essential to clarify your reasons for undertaking this journey. Whether you're seeking to cleanse your body, boost your energy levels, or kickstart healthier habits, defining your intentions can provide motivation and focus throughout the process.

2. **Manage Expectations:** It's important to approach juice detox with realistic expectations. While some people may experience dramatic results, others may notice more subtle changes. Recognize that everyone's experience with detox is unique, and the benefits may manifest differently for each individual.

3. **Address Emotional Support:** Detoxifying the body can sometimes trigger emotional responses as well. Be prepared to address any emotional challenges that may arise during the detox process. Seek support from friends, family, or a professional counselor if needed to navigate through any emotional hurdles.

4. **Practice Mindfulness:** Incorporating mindfulness practices such as meditation, deep breathing exercises, or yoga can help cultivate a positive mindset and reduce stress during the detox period. Mindfulness techniques can also enhance your awareness of bodily sensations and promote a deeper connection with the detox process.

Physical Preparation

1. **Gradual Transition:** Ease into the detox process by gradually reducing your intake of processed foods, caffeine, alcohol, and other potential toxins in the days leading up to the detox. This can help minimize withdrawal symptoms and prepare your body for the transition to a liquid diet.

2. **Stay Hydrated:** Proper hydration is essential for supporting the body's detoxification processes. Start increasing your water intake several days before the detox to ensure that your body is adequately hydrated. Herbal teas and electrolyte-rich beverages can also be beneficial for maintaining hydration levels.

3. **Stock Up on Supplies:** Plan ahead and stock up on fresh fruits and vegetables for juicing, as well as any additional ingredients or supplements you may need during the detox. Investing in a quality juicer or blender can make the juicing process more convenient and enjoyable.

4. **Listen to Your Body:** Pay attention to how your body responds to different foods and beverages leading up to the detox. Notice any food sensitivities or digestive issues that may arise, and make adjustments to your diet as needed to support your overall well-being.

Conclusion

Preparing mentally and physically for a juice detox is essential for setting the stage for a successful and rewarding experience. By clarifying your intentions, managing expectations, and addressing emotional support, you can cultivate a positive mindset and attitude towards the detox process. Gradually transitioning your diet, staying hydrated, and stocking up on supplies can help ensure that your body is adequately prepared for the detox journey. Above all, listen to your body's signals and make adjustments as needed to support your overall health and well-being throughout the detox process.

CHAPTER FIVE

Essential Ingredients: Exploring Detoxifying Herbs, Fruits, and Vegetables

When embarking on a juice detox, selecting the right ingredients is crucial for supporting the body's natural detoxification processes and promoting overall health and well-being. Incorporating a variety of detoxifying herbs, fruits, and vegetables into your juice recipes can help maximize the benefits of the detox and enhance your overall experience. Let's explore some essential ingredients commonly used in juice detox and their detoxifying properties:

1. Leafy Greens:

Leafy greens such as kale, spinach, Swiss chard, and collard greens are nutritional powerhouses rich in chlorophyll, vitamins, minerals, and antioxidants. Chlorophyll, the pigment that gives greens their vibrant color, is known for its detoxifying properties and its ability to support liver health. Leafy greens also contain high levels of fiber, which aids in digestion and promotes regularity, essential for eliminating toxins from the body.

2. Citrus Fruits:

Citrus fruits like lemons, limes, oranges, and grapefruits are excellent additions to juice detox recipes due to their high vitamin C content and alkalizing properties. Vitamin C is a potent antioxidant that helps neutralize free radicals and support immune function. Citrus fruits also have natural diuretic properties, which can help flush out toxins and promote kidney health.

3. Cucumber:

Cucumber is a hydrating and refreshing vegetable that is often included in juice detox recipes for its high water content and cooling properties. Cucumbers are also rich in antioxidants, vitamins, and minerals, including vitamin K, potassium, and magnesium. Their mild flavor makes them an excellent base for green juices and helps balance the stronger flavors of leafy greens and herbs.

4. Ginger:

Ginger is a potent root with anti-inflammatory and digestive properties that can enhance the detoxifying effects of your juices. It contains bioactive compounds such as gingerol and shogaol, which have been shown to support gastrointestinal health, reduce nausea, and alleviate digestive discomfort. Adding fresh ginger to your juice recipes can impart a spicy kick and promote overall digestive wellness.

5. Turmeric:

Turmeric is a bright yellow spice prized for its anti-inflammatory and antioxidant properties, primarily due to its active compound curcumin. Curcumin has been shown to support liver health, aid in detoxification, and reduce inflammation throughout the body. Including fresh turmeric root or powdered turmeric in your juice recipes can add a vibrant color and potent health benefits.

6. Parsley:

Parsley is an herb that packs a nutritional punch, containing vitamins A, C, and K, as well as minerals like potassium and calcium. It is also rich in chlorophyll and flavonoids, which have antioxidant and anti-inflammatory properties. Parsley is often used in juice detox recipes to support kidney health, promote detoxification, and freshen breath.

7. Beets:

Beets are root vegetables known for their vibrant color and impressive nutritional profile. They contain betalains, pigments with antioxidant and anti-inflammatory properties that support liver detoxification and help purify the blood. Beets are also rich in nitrates, which can improve blood flow and cardiovascular health. Including beetroot in your juice recipes can add sweetness and depth of flavor while boosting detoxification.

Conclusion

Incorporating detoxifying herbs, fruits, and vegetables into your juice detox recipes can enhance the cleansing and rejuvenating effects of the detox process. Leafy greens, citrus fruits, cucumber, ginger, turmeric, parsley, and beets are just a few examples of essential ingredients that can support liver health, aid in digestion, reduce inflammation, and promote overall well-being. Experiment with different combinations and flavors to create delicious and nutritious juices that nourish your body and support your detox journey.

CHAPTER SIX

Day 1: Cleansing Juice Recipes for Kickstarting Detoxification

Embarking on a juice detox journey requires careful planning, especially when it comes to selecting the right juice recipes to kickstart the detoxification process. Day 1 sets the tone for the rest of the detox, so it's essential to choose recipes that are both cleansing and nourishing, providing your body with the nutrients it needs to thrive. Below are three cleansing juice recipes designed to kickstart detoxification on Day 1:

1. Green Cleanse Juice:

This vibrant green juice is packed with detoxifying ingredients like leafy greens, cucumber, and lemon, making it an ideal choice for kickstarting your detoxification journey.

Ingredients:

- 2 cups kale leaves

- 1 cucumber

- 1 green apple

- 1/2 lemon (peeled)

- 1-inch piece of ginger

- 1 handful of fresh parsley

Instructions:

1. Wash all the ingredients thoroughly.

2. Peel the lemon and ginger.

3. Cut the cucumber and apple into smaller pieces.

4. Add all the ingredients to a juicer and process until smooth.

5. Pour the juice into a glass and enjoy immediately.

2. Citrus Detox Blast:

This refreshing citrus juice is bursting with vitamin C and antioxidants, making it a perfect choice for cleansing and rejuvenating your body on Day 1 of your detox.

Ingredients:

- 2 oranges (peeled)

- 1 grapefruit (peeled)

- 1 lemon (peeled)

- 1-inch piece of turmeric (or 1/2 tsp turmeric powder)

- 1 carrot (optional, for added sweetness)

Instructions:

1. Peel the oranges, grapefruit, and lemon.

2. Cut the turmeric and carrot into smaller pieces.

3. Add all the ingredients to a juicer and process until well combined.

4. Pour the juice into a glass and enjoy immediately.

3. Beet & Berry Cleanser:

This vibrant juice combines the detoxifying power of beets with the antioxidant-rich goodness of berries, creating a delicious and nutrient-packed drink to jumpstart your detox journey.

Ingredients:

- 1 medium beet (peeled)

- 1 cup mixed berries (such as strawberries, blueberries, and raspberries)

- 1/2 cucumber

- 1/2 lemon (peeled)

- 1-inch piece of ginger

Instructions:

1. Peel the beet and lemon.

2. Cut the beet, cucumber, and lemon into smaller pieces.

3. Add all the ingredients to a juicer and process until smooth.

4. Pour the juice into a glass and enjoy immediately.

Tips for Day 1:

- Start your day with a glass of warm lemon water to hydrate and alkalize your body.

- Sip your juices slowly and mindfully, allowing your body to absorb the nutrients and supporting the detoxification process.

- Stay hydrated throughout the day by drinking plenty of water and herbal teas.

- Listen to your body and adjust the recipes as needed based on your preferences and individual needs.

By incorporating these cleansing juice recipes into your Day 1 of the detox, you can jumpstart your journey towards detoxification, cleansing, and rejuvenation. Remember to stay committed to your goals and embrace the process with an open mind and positive attitude.

CHAPTER SEVEN

Day 2: Nourishing Juices for Continued Detoxification and Energy Replenishment

As you progress through your juice detox journey, Day 2 is an opportunity to continue supporting your body's detoxification process while replenishing energy levels and nourishing your system with vital nutrients. These nourishing juice recipes are designed to provide a boost of energy and sustain you through the second day of your detox:

1. Tropical Green Refresher:

This invigorating green juice combines the refreshing flavors of tropical fruits with the detoxifying properties of leafy greens, providing a burst of energy and essential nutrients to kickstart your day.

Ingredients:

- 1 cup spinach

- 1/2 cup pineapple chunks

- 1/2 cup mango chunks

- 1 kiwi (peeled)

- 1/2 cucumber

- 1/2 lime (peeled)

- 1-inch piece of ginger

Instructions:

1. Wash all the ingredients thoroughly.

2. Peel the lime and ginger.

3. Cut the cucumber and kiwi into smaller pieces.

4. Add all the ingredients to a juicer and process until smooth.

5. Pour the juice into a glass and enjoy immediately.

2. Berry Beet Bliss:

This vibrant red juice combines the detoxifying power of beets with the antioxidant-rich goodness of berries, providing a delicious and nourishing drink to support your detoxification journey.

Ingredients:

- 1 medium beet (peeled)
- 1 cup mixed berries (such as strawberries, blueberries, and raspberries)
- 1/2 cup cucumber
- 1/2 lemon (peeled)
- 1/2 orange (peeled)

- 1-inch piece of ginger

Instructions:

1. Peel the beet, lemon, and orange.

2. Cut the beet, cucumber, lemon, and orange into smaller pieces.

3. Add all the ingredients to a juicer and process until well combined.

4. Pour the juice into a glass and enjoy immediately.

3. Carrot Apple Energizer:

This refreshing juice combines the sweetness of carrots and apples with the zing of ginger, providing a natural energy boost and supporting your body's detoxification efforts.

Ingredients:

- 2 large carrots

- 2 apples (any variety)

- 1/2 lemon (peeled)

- 1-inch piece of ginger

Instructions:

1. Wash all the ingredients thoroughly.

2. Peel the lemon and ginger.

3. Cut the carrots and apples into smaller pieces.

4. Add all the ingredients to a juicer and process until smooth.

5. Pour the juice into a glass and enjoy immediately.

Tips for Day 2:

- Drink your juices slowly and mindfully, allowing your body to absorb the nutrients and sustain energy levels throughout the day.

- Stay hydrated by drinking plenty of water and herbal teas between juices to support the detoxification process.

- Incorporate light physical activity such as walking, yoga, or stretching to promote circulation and enhance detoxification.

- Listen to your body and adjust the recipes as needed based on your preferences and individual needs.

By incorporating these nourishing juice recipes into your Day 2 of the detox, you can continue to support detoxification, replenish energy levels, and nourish your body with essential nutrients. Remember to stay committed to your goals and embrace the process with an open mind and positive attitude.

CHAPTER EIGHT

Day 3: Revitalizing Juices to Wrap Up the Detox and Rejuvenate

As you approach the final day of your juice detox journey, Day 3 is an opportunity to revitalize your body, mind, and spirit with rejuvenating juices that support detoxification and promote overall well-being. These revitalizing juice recipes are designed to provide a final boost of nourishment and leave you feeling refreshed and rejuvenated:

1. Green Revival Elixir:

This green juice combines detoxifying leafy greens with refreshing cucumber and lemon, providing a revitalizing elixir to support your body's natural detoxification processes and promote alkalinity.

Ingredients:

- 2 cups spinach

- 1 cucumber

- 2 celery stalks

- 1 green apple

- 1/2 lemon (peeled)

- 1-inch piece of ginger

Instructions:

1. Wash all the ingredients thoroughly.

2. Peel the lemon and ginger.

3. Cut the cucumber, celery, and apple into smaller pieces.

4. Add all the ingredients to a juicer and process until smooth.

5. Pour the juice into a glass and enjoy immediately.

2. Citrus Sunshine Boost:

This vibrant citrus juice combines the invigorating flavors of oranges, grapefruits, and lemons with the warmth of ginger, providing a burst of energy and vitality to uplift your spirits on the final day of your detox.

Ingredients:

- 2 oranges (peeled)
- 1 grapefruit (peeled)
- 1 lemon (peeled)
- 1-inch piece of ginger

Instructions:

1. Peel the oranges, grapefruit, and lemon.

2. Cut the ginger into smaller pieces.

3. Add all the ingredients to a juicer and process until well combined.

4. Pour the juice into a glass and enjoy immediately.

3. Berry Beet Rejuvenator:

This vibrant red juice combines the detoxifying power of beets with the antioxidant-rich goodness of berries, providing a refreshing and rejuvenating drink to nourish your body and promote overall well-being.

Ingredients:

- 1 medium beet (peeled)
- 1 cup mixed berries (such as strawberries, blueberries, and raspberries)
- 1/2 cucumber
- 1/2 lemon (peeled)
- 1-inch piece of ginger

Instructions:

1. Peel the beet and lemon.

2. Cut the beet, cucumber, and lemon into smaller pieces.

3. Add all the ingredients to a juicer and process until smooth.

4. Pour the juice into a glass and enjoy immediately.

Tips for Day 3:

- Reflect on your detox journey and celebrate your accomplishments, no matter how small. Acknowledge the effort and dedication you've put into nourishing your body and supporting your well-being.

- Take time to rest and relax, allowing your body to fully absorb the benefits of the detox and integrate the nourishment from the juices.

- Gradually reintroduce solid foods into your diet after completing the detox, focusing on whole, nutrient-dense foods to maintain the benefits of the detox and support long-term health.

By incorporating these revitalizing juice recipes into your Day 3 of the detox, you can wrap up your journey on a high note, feeling refreshed, rejuvenated, and ready to embrace a healthier lifestyle. Remember to listen to your body, honor your needs, and celebrate your achievements as you continue on your path towards optimal health and well-being.

CHAPTER NINE

Integrating Juice Detox into Your Lifestyle: Tips for Success

Embarking on a juice detox can be a transformative experience, but integrating it into your lifestyle in a sustainable way is key to long-term success. Whether you're looking to incorporate occasional juice cleanses into your routine or adopt a more permanent lifestyle change, these tips can help you make the most of your juice detox journey:

1. Set Realistic Goals:

- Define clear and achievable goals for your juice detox journey, whether it's to kickstart healthier habits, support weight loss, or improve overall well-being.

- Break down your goals into smaller, actionable steps to help you stay focused and motivated throughout the detox process.

2. Plan Ahead:

- Take time to plan your juice detox journey in advance, including selecting recipes, shopping for ingredients, and scheduling your detox days around your calendar.

- Consider factors such as your work schedule, social commitments, and physical activity level when planning your detox to ensure a smooth and successful experience.

3. Listen to Your Body:

- Pay attention to how your body responds to the juice detox and make adjustments as needed based on your individual needs and preferences.

- If you experience any adverse reactions or discomfort during the detox, consult with a healthcare professional and consider modifying your approach to better suit your body.

4. Stay Hydrated:

- Hydration is crucial during a juice detox, so be sure to drink plenty of water throughout the day to support your body's natural detoxification processes and prevent dehydration.

- Incorporate herbal teas, coconut water, and electrolyte-rich beverages to maintain hydration levels and replenish essential nutrients.

5. Support Your Detox:

- Enhance the detoxification process by incorporating supportive practices such as dry brushing, infrared sauna sessions, or gentle exercise to promote circulation and lymphatic drainage.

- Practice mindfulness techniques such as meditation, deep breathing exercises, or journaling to reduce stress, enhance relaxation, and support overall well-being.

6. Focus on Whole Foods:

- After completing your juice detox, focus on incorporating whole, nutrient-dense foods into your diet to maintain the benefits of the detox and support long-term health.

- Aim to include a variety of fruits, vegetables, whole grains, lean proteins, and healthy fats in your meals to nourish your body and promote optimal wellness.

7. Embrace Balance:

- Find a balance that works for you by incorporating juice detoxes into your lifestyle in a way that feels sustainable and enjoyable.

- Allow yourself flexibility and permission to indulge occasionally while maintaining a foundation of healthy eating habits and self-care practices.

8. Seek Support:

- Surround yourself with a supportive community of friends, family, or like-minded individuals who can offer encouragement, accountability, and guidance throughout your juice detox journey.

- Consider joining online forums, social media groups, or local wellness communities to connect with others who share similar goals and experiences.

By implementing these tips for success, you can integrate juice detox into your lifestyle in a sustainable and empowering way, ultimately supporting your journey towards improved health, vitality, and well-being. Remember that every individual is unique, so it's essential to listen to your body, honor your needs, and adjust your approach as needed to find what works best for you.

CHAPTER TEN

Beyond the 3 Days: Maintaining Detox Results and Incorporating Healthy Habits

Completing a 3-day juice detox can be an empowering experience, but maintaining the results and incorporating healthy habits into your daily routine is essential for long-term success. By continuing to prioritize your health and well-being, you can build upon the foundation established during the detox and cultivate a lifestyle that supports optimal vitality and vitality. Here's how to maintain detox results and incorporate healthy habits beyond the initial 3 days:

1. Gradual Transition:

- Transition back to solid foods gradually after completing the juice detox to prevent digestive discomfort and maintain the benefits of the detox.

- Start with light, easily digestible foods such as fruits, vegetables, soups, and salads before reintroducing heavier or processed foods into your diet.

2. Whole Foods Diet:

- Focus on incorporating whole, nutrient-dense foods into your diet, including a variety of fruits, vegetables, whole grains, lean proteins, and healthy fats.

- Aim to eat a rainbow of colorful fruits and vegetables to ensure a diverse intake of vitamins, minerals, and antioxidants that support overall health and well-being.

3. Hydration:

- Continue to prioritize hydration by drinking plenty of water throughout the day to support detoxification, maintain optimal hydration levels, and promote overall wellness.

- Incorporate hydrating foods such as cucumbers, watermelon, oranges, and leafy greens into your meals and snacks to increase water intake and replenish electrolytes.

4. Balanced Meals:

- Plan balanced meals that include a combination of carbohydrates, protein, and healthy fats to support sustained energy levels, satiety, and overall nutritional needs.

- Choose whole, minimally processed foods whenever possible and avoid excessive consumption of refined sugars, processed foods, and artificial ingredients.

5. Regular Exercise:

- Incorporate regular physical activity into your routine to support overall health, fitness, and well-being.

- Choose activities you enjoy, such as walking, jogging, yoga, swimming, or cycling, and aim for at least 30 minutes of moderate-intensity exercise most days of the week.

6. Mindful Eating:

- Practice mindful eating by paying attention to hunger and fullness cues, eating slowly, and savoring each bite to enhance digestion and promote a healthy relationship with food.

- Minimize distractions while eating, such as watching TV or scrolling on your phone, and focus on the sensory experience of eating to increase satisfaction and enjoyment.

7. Stress Management:

- Prioritize stress management techniques such as meditation, deep breathing exercises, yoga, or mindfulness practices to reduce stress levels, promote relaxation, and support overall well-being.

- Incorporate self-care activities into your daily routine, such as taking regular breaks, spending time outdoors, connecting with loved ones, or engaging in hobbies and interests.

8. Consistency and Persistence:

- Remember that building healthy habits takes time and consistency, so be patient with yourself and stay committed to your health and wellness goals.

- Celebrate your progress, no matter how small, and acknowledge the positive changes you're making towards a healthier lifestyle.

By maintaining detox results and incorporating healthy habits into your daily routine, you can sustain the benefits of your juice detox journey and continue to support your overall health, vitality, and well-being in the long term. Remember to listen to your body, honor your needs, and make choices that align with your values and goals for optimal health and wellness.

Alfalfa:

Definition: Alfalfa, scientifically known as Medicago sativa, is a flowering plant in the pea family native to Asia but cultivated worldwide. It's primarily grown as fodder for livestock, but it has also been used in traditional medicine for its potential health benefits.

Ingredients: Alfalfa contains various bioactive compounds, including vitamins (such as vitamin A, vitamin C, and vitamin K), minerals (including calcium, magnesium, and potassium), amino acids, and phytoestrogens. These compounds are believed to contribute to the herb's medicinal properties, including its potential as a nutritive tonic, diuretic, and hormone balancer.

How to Prepare: Alfalfa is typically consumed as sprouts, herbal tea, or in supplement form (such as capsules or tablets). To make tea, dried alfalfa leaves are steeped in hot water for several minutes before being strained and consumed.

Dosage: The appropriate dosage of alfalfa can vary depending on factors such as age, health status, and the specific preparation being used. It's important to follow the recommended dosage on the product label or consult with a qualified herbalist or healthcare professional for personalized guidance.

How to Use: Alfalfa sprouts, tea, or supplements are typically taken orally. It's often consumed as a dietary supplement to support overall health and well-being, as well as to promote kidney health and hormone balance.

Side Effects: Alfalfa is generally considered safe for most people when consumed in moderate amounts. However, some individuals may experience allergic reactions or digestive upset. It may also interact with certain medications or have adverse effects in individuals with certain health conditions, such as autoimmune diseases or hormone-sensitive conditions. Pregnant or breastfeeding individuals should consult with a healthcare professional before using alfalfa supplements. It's important to use alfalfa under the guidance of a healthcare professional and to discontinue use if any adverse effects occur.

BONUS: SOME HERBAL REMEDIES YOU SHOULD KNOW

Ashwagandha:

Definition: Ashwagandha, scientifically known as Withaniasomnifera, is a small shrub native to India, the Middle East, and parts of Africa. It has a long history of use in Ayurvedic medicine for its potential health benefits, particularly for its adaptogenic properties.

Ingredients: Ashwagandha root contains various bioactive compounds, including alkaloids (such as withanolides), steroidal lactones, and flavonoids. These compounds are believed to contribute to the herb's medicinal properties, including its potential as an adaptogen, anti-inflammatory, and immune-modulating agent.

How to Prepare: Ashwagandha is typically consumed as a powdered root, herbal tea, tincture, or in supplement form (such as capsules or tablets). To make tea, dried ashwagandha root is steeped in hot water for several minutes before being strained and consumed.

Dosage: The appropriate dosage of ashwagandha can vary depending on factors such as age, health status, and the specific preparation being used. It's important to follow the recommended dosage on the product label or consult with a qualified herbalist or healthcare professional for personalized guidance.

How to Use: Ashwagandha powder, tea, tincture, or supplements are typically taken orally. It's often consumed to support stress management, promote relaxation, and boost overall vitality and well-being.

Side Effects: Ashwagandha is generally considered safe for most people when used in moderate amounts. However, some individuals may experience mild side effects such as gastrointestinal upset or drowsiness. It may also interact with certain medications or have adverse effects in individuals with certain health conditions, such as autoimmune diseases or thyroid disorders. Pregnant or breastfeeding individuals should consult with a healthcare professional before using ashwagandha supplements. It's important to use ashwagandha under the guidance of a healthcare professional and to discontinue use if any adverse effects occur.

Cat's Claw:

Definition: Cat's claw, scientifically known as Uncaria tomentosa, is a woody vine native to the Amazon rainforest and other parts of Central and South America. It has been used for centuries in traditional medicine by indigenous peoples for its potential health benefits.

Ingredients: Cat's claw contains various bioactive compounds, including alkaloids (such as oxindole alkaloids and quinovic acid glycosides), polyphenols, and other phytochemicals. These compounds are believed to contribute to the herb's medicinal properties, including its potential as an immune enhancer, anti-inflammatory, and antioxidant.

How to Prepare: Cat's claw is typically consumed as an herbal tea, tincture, or in supplement form (such as capsules or tablets). To make tea, dried cat's claw bark or leaves are steeped in hot water for several minutes before being strained and consumed.

Dosage: The appropriate dosage of cat's claw can vary depending on factors such as age, health status, and the specific preparation being used. It's important to follow the recommended dosage on the product label or consult with a qualified herbalist or healthcare professional for personalized guidance.

How to Use: Cat's claw tea, tincture, or supplements are typically taken orally. It's often used to support immune function, reduce inflammation, and promote overall well-being.

Side Effects: Cat's claw is generally considered safe for most people when used in moderate amounts. However, some individuals may experience mild side effects such as gastrointestinal upset or allergic reactions. It may also interact with certain medications or have adverse effects in individuals with certain health conditions, such as autoimmune diseases or bleeding disorders. Pregnant or breastfeeding individuals should consult with a healthcare professional before using cat's claw supplements. It's important to use cat's claw under the guidance of a healthcare professional and to discontinue use if any adverse effects occur.

Chickweed:

Definition: Chickweed, scientifically known as Stellaria media, is an annual herbaceous plant native to Europe but naturalized in many other parts of the world. It's often considered a common weed but has been used historically in traditional medicine for its potential health benefits.

Ingredients: Chickweed contains various bioactive compounds, including flavonoids, saponins, mucilage, and vitamins (such as vitamin C). These compounds are believed to contribute to the herb's medicinal properties, including its potential as a demulcent, anti-inflammatory, and mild diuretic.

How to Prepare: Chickweed is typically consumed as an herbal tea, infusion, or in fresh salads. To make tea, dried chickweed leaves and flowers are steeped in hot water for several minutes before being strained and consumed. It can also be used topically as a poultice or infused oil for skin conditions.

Dosage: The appropriate dosage of chickweed can vary depending on factors such as age, health status, and the specific preparation being used. It's important to follow the recommended dosage on the product label or consult with a qualified herbalist or healthcare professional for personalized guidance.

How to Use: Chickweed tea, infusion, or fresh leaves are typically taken orally. It's often used to soothe inflammation, support digestion, and promote overall well-being. Topically, chickweed can be applied to the skin to alleviate itching, irritation, or minor wounds.

Side Effects: Chickweed is generally considered safe for most people when consumed in moderate amounts. However, some individuals may experience allergic reactions or gastrointestinal upset. It may also interact with certain medications or have adverse effects in individuals with certain health conditions. Pregnant or breastfeeding individuals should consult with a healthcare professional before using chickweed supplements. It's important to use chickweed under the guidance of a healthcare professional and to discontinue use if any adverse effects occur.

Cleavers:

Definition: Cleavers, scientifically known as Galium aparine, is a herbaceous annual plant native to Europe, North America, Asia, and Australia. It has a long history of use in traditional medicine for its potential health benefits.

Ingredients: Cleavers contains various bioactive compounds, including iridoid glycosides, flavonoids, tannins, and mucilage. These compounds are believed to contribute to the herb's medicinal properties, including its potential as a diuretic, lymphatic tonic, and mild astringent.

How to Prepare: Cleavers is typically consumed as an herbal tea, infusion, or in fresh salads. To make tea, dried cleavers leaves and stems are steeped in hot water for several minutes before being strained and consumed. It can also be used topically as a poultice or infused oil for skin conditions.

Dosage: The appropriate dosage of cleavers can vary depending on factors such as age, health status, and the specific preparation being used. It's important to follow the recommended dosage on the product label or consult with a qualified herbalist or healthcare professional for personalized guidance.

How to Use: Cleavers tea, infusion, or fresh leaves are typically taken orally. It's often used to support lymphatic drainage, promote urinary tract health, and soothe inflammation. Topically, cleavers can be applied to the skin to alleviate itching, irritation, or minor wounds.

Side Effects: Cleavers is generally considered safe for most people when consumed in moderate amounts. However, some individuals may experience allergic reactions or gastrointestinal upset. It may also interact with certain medications or have adverse effects in individuals with certain health conditions. Pregnant or breastfeeding individuals should consult with a healthcare professional before using cleavers supplements. It's important to use cleavers under the guidance of a healthcare professional and to discontinue use if any adverse effects occur.

Eucalyptus:

Definition: Eucalyptus refers to a genus of flowering trees and shrubs, primarily native to Australia but also found in other parts of the world. Eucalyptus essential oil, extracted from the leaves of certain species, has a long history of use in traditional medicine for its potential health benefits.

Ingredients: Eucalyptus essential oil contains various bioactive compounds, including eucalyptol (cineole), terpenes, and flavonoids. These compounds are believed to contribute to the oil's medicinal properties, including its potential as an expectorant, decongestant, antiseptic, and anti-inflammatory.

How to Prepare: Eucalyptus essential oil can be used in aromatherapy, diffused in the air, or diluted and applied topically to the skin. It can also be added to steam inhalations or chest rubs to help relieve respiratory symptoms.

Dosage: The appropriate dosage of eucalyptus essential oil can vary depending on factors such as age, health status, and the specific application being used. It's important to follow the recommended dosage on the product label or consult with a qualified aromatherapist or healthcare professional for personalized guidance.

How to Use: Eucalyptus essential oil can be used aromatically, topically, or internally, depending on the intended application. It's often used to alleviate respiratory congestion, soothe sore muscles, promote relaxation, and support overall well-being.

Side Effects: Eucalyptus essential oil is generally considered safe for most people when used appropriately. However, it can be toxic if ingested in large amounts and should not be applied directly to the skin without proper dilution. Some individuals may experience allergic reactions or respiratory irritation when exposed to eucalyptus oil. It's important to use eucalyptus oil with caution, especially around children and pets. Pregnant or breastfeeding individuals should consult with a healthcare professional before using eucalyptus oil. If any adverse effects occur, discontinue use and seek medical attention.

Feverfew:

Definition: Feverfew, scientifically known as Tanacetum parthenium, is a perennial herb native to Europe but also found in other parts of the world. It has a long history of use in traditional medicine, particularly in European folk medicine, for its potential health benefits.

Ingredients: Feverfew contains various bioactive compounds, including sesquiterpene lactones (such as parthenolide), flavonoids, and volatile oils. These compounds are believed to contribute to the herb's medicinal properties, including its potential as an anti-inflammatory, analgesic, and migraine prophylactic.

How to Prepare: Feverfew is typically consumed as an herbal tea, tincture, or in supplement form (such as capsules or tablets). To make tea, dried feverfew leaves and flowers are steeped in hot water for several minutes before being strained and consumed.

Dosage: The appropriate dosage of feverfew can vary depending on factors such as age, health status, and the specific preparation being used. It's important to follow the recommended dosage on the product label or consult with a qualified herbalist or healthcare professional for personalized guidance.

How to Use: Feverfew tea, tincture, or supplements are typically taken orally. It's often used to alleviate headaches, including migraines, and to support overall well-being.

Side Effects: Feverfew is generally considered safe for most people when used in moderate amounts. However, some individuals may experience mild side effects such as gastrointestinal upset or allergic reactions. It may also interact with certain medications or have adverse effects in individuals with certain health conditions, such as bleeding disorders or pregnancy. It's important to use feverfew under the guidance of a healthcare professional and to discontinue use if any adverse effects occur.

Ginseng:

Definition: Ginseng refers to several species of perennial plants belonging to the Panax genus, including Panax ginseng (Asian ginseng) and Panax quinquefolius (American ginseng). Ginseng has been used for centuries in traditional medicine, particularly in East Asia, for its potential health benefits.

Ingredients: Ginseng root contains various bioactive compounds, including ginsenosides, polysaccharides, and peptides. These compounds are believed to contribute to the herb's medicinal properties, including its potential as an adaptogen, immune enhancer, and cognitive booster.

How to Prepare: Ginseng is typically consumed as a powdered root, herbal tea, tincture, or in supplement form (such as capsules or tablets). To make tea, dried ginseng root slices are simmered in water for several minutes before being strained and consumed.

Dosage: The appropriate dosage of ginseng can vary depending on factors such as age, health status, and the specific preparation being used. It's important to follow the recommended dosage on the product label or consult with a qualified herbalist or healthcare professional for personalized guidance.

How to Use: Ginseng powder, tea, tincture, or supplements are typically taken orally. It's often used to support energy levels, enhance cognitive function, and promote overall well-being.

Side Effects: Ginseng is generally considered safe for most people when used in moderate amounts. However, some individuals may experience mild side effects such as insomnia, gastrointestinal upset, or headaches. It may also interact with certain medications or have adverse effects in individuals with certain health conditions, such as high blood pressure or diabetes. Pregnant or breastfeeding individuals should consult with a healthcare professional before using ginseng supplements. It's important to use ginseng under the guidance of a healthcare professional and to discontinue use if any adverse effects occur.

Bio Ferro Tonic:

Definition: Bio Ferro Tonic is a dietary supplement primarily composed of herbs and minerals. It's often marketed as a natural way to support overall health, particularly by promoting blood health and circulation.

Ingredients: Typical ingredients in Bio Ferro Tonic may include a blend of herbs such as burdock root, yellow dock root, sarsaparilla root, and cascara sagrada bark, along with minerals like iron and potassium phosphate.

How to Prepare: Bio Ferro Tonic usually comes in liquid form and is typically taken orally. It's important to follow the instructions on the product label for dosage and administration.

Dosage: The dosage can vary depending on the specific product and individual needs. It's crucial to consult with a healthcare professional or follow the recommended dosage on the product label to avoid potential side effects.

How to Use: Bio Ferro Tonic is often taken by adding the recommended dosage to water or juice and consuming it orally. It's important to shake the bottle well before use and store it according to the manufacturer's instructions.

Side Effects: While Bio Ferro Tonic is generally considered safe when used as directed, some individuals may experience side effects such as digestive discomfort, allergic reactions, or interactions with medications. It's essential to consult with a healthcare provider before starting any new supplement regimen, especially if you have underlying health conditions or are taking medications.

Bladderwrack:

Definition: Bladderwrack is a type of seaweed or marine algae commonly used in traditional medicine and as a dietary supplement. It's known for its potential health benefits, particularly related to thyroid health and weight management.

Ingredients: Bladderwrack contains various nutrients, including iodine, vitamins, minerals, and antioxidants. The primary active components are iodine and fucoidan, a type of carbohydrate found in brown seaweeds.

How to Prepare: Bladderwrack supplements are available in various forms, including capsules, powders, and liquid extracts. They can be taken orally with water or added to smoothies and other beverages.

Dosage: The appropriate dosage of bladderwrack can vary based on factors such as age, health status, and the specific product being used. It's essential to follow the recommended dosage on the product label or consult with a healthcare professional for personalized guidance.

How to Use: Bladderwrack supplements are typically taken orally, either with water or mixed into food or beverages. It's important to follow the instructions on the product label and avoid exceeding the recommended dosage.

Side Effects: While bladderwrack is generally considered safe for most people when used in moderation, excessive intake of iodine from bladderwrack supplements can cause thyroid dysfunction and other adverse effects. Individuals with thyroid disorders, iodine sensitivity, or certain medical conditions should exercise caution and consult with a healthcare provider before using bladderwrack supplements. Common side effects may include digestive upset, allergic reactions, or interactions with medications.

Blood Purifier:

Definition: Blood purifiers are herbal remedies or dietary supplements believed to cleanse or detoxify the blood, often promoting overall health and well-being. They are thought to support the body's natural detoxification processes and improve blood circulation.

Ingredients: Blood purifiers may contain a variety of herbs and botanical extracts known for their purported cleansing and detoxifying properties. Common ingredients include burdock root, red clover, dandelion root, and yellow dock root, among others.

How to Prepare: Blood purifiers are typically available in various forms, including capsules, tablets, powders, and liquid extracts. They are usually taken orally with water or juice, following the recommended dosage on the product label.

Dosage: The dosage of blood purifiers can vary depending on the specific product and individual needs. It's important to adhere to the recommended dosage on the product label or consult with a healthcare professional for personalized guidance.

How to Use: Blood purifiers are typically taken orally, either with water or mixed into beverages. They are often used as part of a detoxification regimen or to support overall health and vitality.

Side Effects: While blood purifiers are generally considered safe for most people when used as directed, some individuals may experience side effects such as digestive discomfort, allergic reactions, or interactions with medications. It's important to consult with a healthcare provider before starting any new supplement regimen, especially if you have underlying health conditions or are taking medications.

Blue Vervain:

Definition: Blue vervain, also known as Verbena hastata, is a perennial herb native to North America. It has been used in traditional medicine for centuries to treat various ailments, including anxiety, insomnia, and digestive issues.

Ingredients: Blue vervain contains several active compounds, including aucubin, verbenalin, and volatile oils. These compounds are believed to contribute to the herb's medicinal properties.

How to Prepare: Blue vervain is typically consumed as a tea or tincture. To make tea, dried blue vervain leaves and flowers are steeped in hot water for several minutes before being strained and consumed. Tinctures are prepared by steeping the herb in alcohol or vinegar to extract its active compounds.

Dosage: The appropriate dosage of blue vervain can vary depending on factors such as age, health status, and the specific preparation being used. It's important to follow the recommended dosage on the product label or consult with a qualified herbalist or healthcare professional for personalized guidance.

How to Use: Blue vervain tea or tincture is typically taken orally. It can be consumed on its own or mixed with honey or other herbal teas for added flavor.

Side Effects: While blue vervain is generally considered safe for most people when used in moderation, excessive intake may cause digestive upset or allergic reactions in some individuals. Pregnant or breastfeeding women should avoid blue vervain due to its potential to stimulate uterine contractions. As with any herbal remedy, it's important to consult with a healthcare provider before using blue vervain, especially if you have underlying health conditions or are taking medications.

Bromide Plus Powder:

Definition: Bromide Plus Powder is a dietary supplement formulated to support thyroid health and promote overall well-being. It typically contains a blend of herbs and minerals that are believed to have beneficial effects on thyroid function.

Ingredients: Bromide Plus Powder often contains a combination of herbs such as bladderwrack, sea moss, and burdock root, along with minerals like iodine and potassium phosphate. These ingredients are thought to support thyroid function and maintain optimal iodine levels in the body.

How to Prepare: Bromide Plus Powder is usually mixed with water or juice to create a drinkable solution. It's important to follow the instructions on the product label for dosage and preparation.

Dosage: The dosage of Bromide Plus Powder can vary depending on the specific product and individual needs. It's crucial to consult with a healthcare professional or follow the recommended dosage on the product label to avoid potential side effects.

How to Use: Bromide Plus Powder is typically taken orally by mixing the recommended dosage with water or juice. It's important to shake or stir the mixture well before consuming it to ensure even distribution of the ingredients.

Side Effects: While Bromide Plus Powder is generally considered safe when used as directed, some individuals may experience side effects such as digestive discomfort or allergic reactions to certain ingredients. It's essential to consult with a healthcare provider before starting any new supplement regimen, especially if you have underlying health conditions or are taking medications.

Bugleweed:

Definition: Bugleweed, also known as Lycopusvirginicus, is a perennial herb native to North America and Europe. It has been used in traditional medicine to treat various conditions, including hyperthyroidism, anxiety, and insomnia.

Ingredients: Bugleweed contains several active compounds, including lithospermic acid, phenolic acids, and flavonoids. These compounds are believed to contribute to the herb's medicinal properties, particularly its ability to regulate thyroid function.

How to Prepare: Bugleweed is commonly consumed as a tea or tincture. To make tea, dried bugleweed leaves and flowers are steeped in hot water for several minutes before being strained and consumed. Tinctures are prepared by steeping the herb in alcohol or vinegar to extract its active compounds.

Dosage: The appropriate dosage of bugleweed can vary depending on factors such as age, health status, and the specific preparation being used. It's important to follow the recommended dosage on the product label or consult with a qualified herbalist or healthcare professional for personalized guidance.

How to Use: Bugleweed tea or tincture is typically taken orally. It can be consumed on its own or mixed with honey or other herbal teas for added flavor.

Side Effects: While bugleweed is generally considered safe for most people when used in moderation, excessive intake may cause digestive upset or allergic reactions in some individuals. Pregnant or breastfeeding women should avoid bugleweed due to its potential to stimulate uterine contractions. As with any herbal remedy, it's important to consult with a healthcare provider before using bugleweed, especially if you have underlying health conditions or are taking medications.

Burdock:

Definition: Burdock, scientifically known as Arctium lappa, is a biennial plant native to Europe and Asia but now found worldwide. It's part of the Asteraceae family and has been used for centuries in traditional medicine and culinary practices.

Ingredients: Burdock contains various nutrients, including carbohydrates, fiber, vitamins (such as vitamin B6, folate, and vitamin C), and minerals (including potassium, magnesium, and manganese). It also contains active compounds such as polyphenols and volatile oils.

How to Prepare: Burdock can be prepared and consumed in various ways. The roots, leaves, and seeds are all utilized for different purposes. The root is commonly used in cooking, herbal teas, tinctures, and supplements, while the leaves and seeds are sometimes used in herbal preparations.

Dosage: The appropriate dosage of burdock root can vary depending on the specific form and intended use. For culinary purposes, there are no strict dosage guidelines, but for supplements or herbal remedies, it's essential to follow the recommended dosage on the product label or consult with a healthcare professional.

How to Use: Burdock root can be used in cooking by peeling, slicing, and adding it to soups, stews, stir-fries, or salads. It can also be brewed into a tea or used to make tinctures or extracts for medicinal purposes. Some people may also take burdock root supplements in capsule or powder form.

Side Effects: While burdock is generally considered safe for most people when consumed in moderate amounts, some individuals may experience allergic reactions or digestive upset. Additionally, burdock may interact with certain medications or have adverse effects in individuals with certain health conditions, such as diabetes or allergies to plants in the Asteraceae family. It's important to consult with a healthcare provider before using burdock, especially if you have underlying health conditions or are taking medications.

Cascara Sagrada:

Definition: Cascara Sagrada, scientifically known as Rhamnus purshiana, is a species of buckthorn native to western North America. It has been used traditionally as a laxative and to promote bowel regularity.

Ingredients: The primary active ingredients in cascara sagrada are anthraquinone glycosides, particularly cascarosides A and B. These compounds stimulate peristalsis in the colon, leading to increased bowel movements.

How to Prepare: Cascara sagrada is typically prepared as an herbal tea, tincture, or capsule. To make tea, dried cascara sagrada bark is steeped in hot water for several minutes before being strained and consumed. Tinctures are prepared by steeping the bark in alcohol to extract its active compounds.

Dosage: The appropriate dosage of cascara sagrada can vary depending on the specific preparation and intended use. It's important to follow the recommended dosage on the product label or consult with a healthcare professional for personalized guidance.

How to Use: Cascara sagrada tea or tincture is typically taken orally. It's important to start with a low dose and gradually increase if needed to avoid potential side effects such as cramping or diarrhea.

Side Effects: Cascara sagrada is considered safe for short-term use when used as directed. However, long-term or excessive use may lead to dependence, electrolyte imbalance, or dehydration. It may also interact with certain medications or have adverse effects in individuals with certain health conditions. It's important to use cascara sagrada under the guidance of a healthcare professional and to discontinue use if any adverse effects occur.

Cell Food:

Definition: Cell Food is a dietary supplement marketed as a highly oxygenating and alkalizing formula. It's claimed to support overall health and vitality by providing essential nutrients and oxygen to the cells.

Ingredients: The exact ingredients of Cell Food can vary depending on the brand, but it typically contains a proprietary blend of minerals, enzymes, electrolytes, and trace elements. Some common ingredients may include purified water, dissolved oxygen, seawater extract, and plant-based enzymes.

How to Prepare: Cell Food is usually available in liquid form and is typically taken orally. It can be consumed directly or diluted in water or juice before consumption.

Dosage: The dosage of Cell Food can vary depending on the specific product and individual needs. It's important to follow the recommended dosage on the product label or consult with a healthcare professional for personalized guidance.

How to Use: Cell Food is typically taken orally, either directly or mixed into water or juice. It's important to shake the bottle well before use and to store it according to the manufacturer's instructions.

Side Effects: Cell Food is generally considered safe for most people when used as directed. However, some individuals may experience mild digestive upset or allergic reactions to certain ingredients. It's essential to consult with a healthcare provider before starting any new supplement regimen, especially if you have underlying health conditions or are taking medications.

Chaparral:

Definition: Chaparral, scientifically known as Larrea tridentata, is a shrub native to the southwestern United States and northern Mexico. It has been used for centuries by Native American tribes for its medicinal properties and is commonly used in herbal medicine today.

Ingredients: Chaparral contains several bioactive compounds, including nordihydroguaiaretic acid (NDGA), flavonoids, lignans, and volatile oils. NDGA is believed to be the primary active compound responsible for many of chaparral's therapeutic effects.

How to Prepare: Chaparral can be prepared and consumed in various forms, including teas, tinctures, capsules, and topical preparations. To make tea, dried chaparral leaves are steeped in hot water for several minutes before being strained and consumed. Tinctures are prepared by steeping the herb in alcohol or vinegar to extract its active compounds.

Dosage: The appropriate dosage of chaparral can vary depending on the specific form and intended use. It's important to follow the recommended dosage on the product label or consult with a healthcare professional for personalized guidance.

How to Use: Chaparral tea or tincture is typically taken orally. It can also be applied topically to the skin for certain conditions. It's important to use chaparral products as directed and to discontinue use if any adverse effects occur.

Side Effects: Chaparral is generally considered safe for most people when used in moderate amounts. However, excessive intake or prolonged use may lead to liver toxicity or other adverse effects. It may also interact with certain medications or have adverse effects in individuals with certain health conditions. It's important to use chaparral under the guidance of a healthcare professional and to discontinue use if any adverse effects occur.

Dandelion Root:

Definition: Dandelion, scientifically known as Taraxacum officinale, is a common flowering plant found worldwide. While often considered a pesky weed, dandelion has a long history of use in traditional medicine for its various health benefits.

Ingredients: Dandelion root contains several bioactive compounds, including sesquiterpene lactones, triterpenes, flavonoids, and polysaccharides. These compounds are believed to contribute to the herb's medicinal properties, including its potential as a diuretic, digestive aid, and liver tonic.

How to Prepare: Dandelion root can be prepared and consumed in various forms, including teas, tinctures, capsules, and extracts. To make tea, dried dandelion root is steeped in hot water for several minutes before being strained and consumed. Tinctures are prepared by steeping the root in alcohol or vinegar to extract its active compounds.

Dosage: The appropriate dosage of dandelion root can vary depending on factors such as age, health status, and the specific preparation being used. It's important to follow the recommended dosage on the product label or consult with a qualified herbalist or healthcare professional for personalized guidance.

How to Use: Dandelion root tea, tincture, or capsules are typically taken orally. It's important to use dandelion root products as directed and to discontinue use if any adverse effects occur.

Side Effects: Dandelion root is generally considered safe for most people when used in moderate amounts. However, some individuals may experience allergic reactions or digestive upset. It may also interact with certain medications or have adverse effects in individuals with certain health conditions. It's important to use dandelion root under the guidance of a healthcare professional and to discontinue use if any adverse effects occur.

Green Food Plus:

Definition: Green Food Plus is a dietary supplement formulated to provide a concentrated source of nutrients derived from various green plants. It's designed to support overall health and well-being by delivering essential vitamins, minerals, antioxidants, and phytonutrients.

Ingredients: Green Food Plus typically contains a blend of powdered green vegetables, grasses, algae, and other plant-based ingredients. Common ingredients may include wheatgrass, barley grass, spirulina, chlorella, alfalfa, kale, spinach, and broccoli, among others.

How to Prepare: Green Food Plus is usually available in powder form and can be mixed with water, juice, or smoothies. It's important to follow the recommended dosage on the product label and to consume it as part of a balanced diet.

Dosage: The appropriate dosage of Green Food Plus can vary depending on the specific product and individual needs. It's important to follow the recommended dosage on the product label or consult with a healthcare professional for personalized guidance.

How to Use: Green Food Plus powder is typically mixed with water, juice, or smoothies and consumed orally. It's often taken once or twice daily, preferably with meals, to maximize nutrient absorption.

Side Effects: Green Food Plus is generally considered safe for most people when used as directed. However, some individuals may experience digestive upset or allergic reactions to certain ingredients. It's important to consult with a healthcare provider before starting any new supplement regimen, especially if you have underlying health conditions or are taking medications.

Guaco:

Definition: Guaco, also known as Mikania cordata or Mikania glomerata, is a medicinal plant native to Central and South America. It has a long history of use in traditional medicine for its potential therapeutic properties.

Ingredients: Guaco contains several bioactive compounds, including coumarins, flavonoids, tannins, and saponins. These compounds are believed to contribute to the herb's medicinal properties, including its potential as an expectorant, anti-inflammatory, and antispasmodic agent.

How to Prepare: Guaco is typically prepared and consumed as an herbal tea or infusion. To make tea, dried guaco leaves are steeped in hot water for several minutes before being strained and consumed.

Dosage: The appropriate dosage of guaco can vary depending on factors such as age, health status, and the specific preparation being used. It's important to follow the recommended dosage on the product label or consult with a qualified herbalist or healthcare professional for personalized guidance.

How to Use: Guaco tea is typically taken orally. It can be consumed on its own or mixed with honey or other herbal teas for added flavor.

Side Effects: Guaco is generally considered safe for most people when used in moderate amounts. However, some individuals may experience allergic reactions or digestive upset. It may also interact with certain medications or have adverse effects in individuals with certain health conditions. It's important to use guaco under the guidance of a healthcare professional and to discontinue use if any adverse effects occur.

Cocolmeca:

Definition: Cocolmeca, also known as Smilax ornata or sarsaparilla, is a flowering vine native to Mexico and Central America. It has been used traditionally in Mexican and Central American folk medicine for its purported medicinal properties.

Ingredients: Cocolmeca contains various bioactive compounds, including saponins, flavonoids, and plant sterols. These compounds are believed to contribute to the herb's medicinal properties, including its potential as a diuretic, blood purifier, and anti-inflammatory agent.

How to Prepare: Cocolmeca is commonly prepared and consumed as an herbal tea or decoction. To make tea, dried cocolmeca roots or leaves are steeped in hot water for several minutes before being strained and consumed. Decoctions involve boiling the roots or leaves in water to extract their active compounds.

Dosage: The appropriate dosage of cocolmeca can vary depending on factors such as age, health status, and the specific preparation being used. It's important to follow the recommended dosage on the product label or consult with a qualified herbalist or healthcare professional for personalized guidance.

How to Use: Cocolmeca tea or decoction is typically taken orally. It can also be used topically for certain skin conditions. It's important to use cocolmeca products as directed and to discontinue use if any adverse effects occur.

Side Effects: Cocolmeca is generally considered safe for most people when used in moderate amounts. However, excessive intake may lead to digestive upset or other adverse effects. It may also interact with certain medications or have adverse effects in individuals with certain health conditions. It's important to use cocolmeca under the guidance of a healthcare professional and to discontinue use if any adverse effects occur.

Contribo:

Definition: Contribo, also known as Aristolochiatrilobata, is a vine native to the Caribbean and Central America. It has been used traditionally in folk medicine for various purposes, including as a remedy for digestive issues, inflammation, and pain relief.

Ingredients: Contribo contains several bioactive compounds, including aristolochic acids, flavonoids, and alkaloids. These compounds are believed to contribute to the herb's medicinal properties, including its potential as an anti-inflammatory and analgesic agent.

How to Prepare: Contribo is typically prepared and consumed as an herbal tea or decoction. To make tea, dried contribo leaves or stems are steeped in hot water for several minutes before being strained and consumed. Decoctions involve boiling the leaves or stems in water to extract their active compounds.

Dosage: The appropriate dosage of contribo can vary depending on factors such as age, health status, and the specific preparation being used. It's important to follow the recommended dosage on the product label or consult with a qualified herbalist or healthcare professional for personalized guidance.

How to Use: Contribo tea or decoction is typically taken orally. It's important to use contribo products as directed and to discontinue use if any adverse effects occur.

Side Effects: Contribo contains aristolochic acids, which have been associated with serious adverse effects, including kidney damage and cancer. Due to these safety concerns, the use of contribo is highly discouraged, and it's important to avoid products containing aristolochic acids. Individuals should seek alternative remedies for their health needs.

Goldenseal:

Definition: Goldenseal, scientifically known as Hydrastis canadensis, is a perennial herb native to North America. It has a long history of use in traditional Native American medicine and later in folk medicine for its potential health benefits.

Ingredients: Goldenseal root contains various bioactive compounds, including alkaloids (such as berberine and hydrastine), flavonoids, and volatile oils. These compounds are believed to contribute to the herb's medicinal properties, including its potential as an antimicrobial, anti-inflammatory, and immune enhancer.

How to Prepare: Goldenseal is typically consumed as an herbal tea, tincture, or in supplement form (such as capsules or tablets). To make tea, dried goldenseal root or leaves are steeped in hot water for several minutes before being strained and consumed.

Dosage: The appropriate dosage of goldenseal can vary depending on factors such as age, health status, and the specific preparation being used. It's important to follow the recommended dosage on the product label or consult with a qualified herbalist or healthcare professional for personalized guidance.

How to Use: Goldenseal tea, tincture, or supplements are typically taken orally. It's often used to support immune function, promote digestive health, and soothe inflammation.

Side Effects: Goldenseal is generally considered safe for most people when used in moderate amounts. However, some individuals may experience mild side effects such as gastrointestinal upset or allergic reactions. It may also interact with certain medications or have adverse effects in individuals with certain health conditions, such as high blood pressure or pregnancy. It's important to use goldenseal under the guidance of a healthcare professional and to discontinue use if any adverse effects occur.

Hops:

Definition: Hops, scientifically known as Humulus lupulus, is a perennial climbing vine native to Europe, Asia, and North America. It is primarily known for its use in brewing beer but has also been used historically in traditional medicine for its potential health benefits.

Ingredients: Hops flowers contain various bioactive compounds, including bitter acids (such as humulone and lupulone), essential oils, flavonoids, and polyphenols. These compounds are believed to contribute to the herb's medicinal properties, including its potential as a sedative, relaxant, and digestive aid.

How to Prepare: Hops is typically consumed as an herbal tea, tincture, or in supplement form (such as capsules or tablets). To make tea, dried hops flowers are steeped in hot water for several minutes before being strained and consumed.

Dosage: The appropriate dosage of hops can vary depending on factors such as age, health status, and the specific preparation being used. It's important to follow the recommended dosage on the product label or consult with a qualified herbalist or healthcare professional for personalized guidance.

How to Use: Hops tea, tincture, or supplements are typically taken orally. It's often used to promote relaxation, relieve anxiety, and support sleep.

Side Effects: Hops is generally considered safe for most people when used in moderate amounts. However, some individuals may experience mild side effects such as drowsiness, gastrointestinal upset, or allergic reactions. It may also interact with certain medications or have adverse effects in individuals with certain health conditions, such as depression or hormone-sensitive conditions. It's important to use hops under the guidance of a healthcare professional and to discontinue use if any adverse effects occur.

Kelp:

Definition: Kelp refers to several species of large brown algae belonging to the Laminariales order. It is commonly found in underwater forests along rocky coastlines around the world. Kelp has been used for centuries in various cultures, particularly in East Asia, for its nutritional and medicinal properties.

Ingredients: Kelp is rich in various nutrients, including iodine, vitamins (such as vitamin K, vitamin C, and B vitamins), minerals (including calcium, magnesium, and potassium), antioxidants, and fiber. These nutrients are believed to contribute to the seaweed's potential health benefits, including its role in thyroid function, bone health, and immune support.

How to Prepare: Kelp is typically consumed dried, powdered, or in supplement form (such as capsules or tablets). It can also be used in cooking, particularly in soups, salads, and stir-fries. Kelp supplements are available in various forms, including powdered extracts, tablets, and liquid extracts.

Dosage: The appropriate dosage of kelp can vary depending on factors such as age, health status, and the specific preparation being used. It's important to follow the recommended dosage on the product label or consult with a qualified healthcare professional for personalized guidance.

How to Use: Kelp supplements are typically taken orally with water. They can be consumed as part of a daily nutritional regimen to support overall health and well-being. Kelp can also be incorporated into recipes as a flavorful and nutritious ingredient.

Side Effects: While kelp is generally considered safe for most people when consumed in moderate amounts, excessive intake of iodine-rich foods or supplements, including kelp, can lead to thyroid dysfunction or iodine toxicity. Some individuals may also be allergic to seaweed and experience allergic reactions. Pregnant or breastfeeding individuals should consult with a healthcare professional before using kelp supplements. It's important to use kelp under the guidance of a healthcare professional and to discontinue use if any adverse effects occur.

Astragalus:

Definition: Astragalus, scientifically known as Astragalus membranaceus, is a flowering plant native to China and Mongolia but also found in other parts of Asia. It has been used for centuries in traditional Chinese medicine for its potential health benefits, particularly for its immune-enhancing properties.

Ingredients: Astragalus root contains various bioactive compounds, including polysaccharides, saponins (such as astragalosides), flavonoids, and amino acids. These compounds are believed to contribute to the herb's medicinal properties, including its potential as an adaptogen, immunomodulator, and anti-inflammatory agent.

How to Prepare: Astragalus is typically consumed as a powdered root, herbal tea, tincture, or in supplement form (such as capsules or tablets). To make tea, dried astragalus root slices are simmered in water for several minutes before being strained and consumed.

Dosage: The appropriate dosage of astragalus can vary depending on factors such as age, health status, and the specific preparation being used. It's important to follow the recommended dosage on the product label or consult with a qualified herbalist or healthcare professional for personalized guidance.

How to Use: Astragalus powder, tea, tincture, or supplements are typically taken orally. It's often consumed to support immune function, promote vitality, and enhance overall well-being.

Side Effects: Astragalus is generally considered safe for most people when used in moderate amounts. However, some individuals may experience mild side effects such as gastrointestinal upset or allergic reactions. It may also interact with certain medications or have adverse effects in individuals with certain health conditions, such as autoimmune diseases or diabetes. Pregnant or breastfeeding individuals should consult with a healthcare professional before using astragalus supplements. It's important to use astragalus under the guidance of a healthcare professional and to discontinue use if any adverse effects occur.

Black Cohosh:

Definition: Black cohosh, scientifically known as Actaea racemosa (formerly Cimicifuga racemosa), is a perennial herb native to North America. It has a long history of use in traditional Native American medicine and later in folk medicine for its potential health benefits, particularly for women's health.

Ingredients: Black cohosh root contains various bioactive compounds, including triterpene glycosides (such as actein and cimicifugoside), phenolic acids, and flavonoids. These compounds are believed to contribute to the herb's medicinal properties, including its potential as a hormone-balancing agent and its ability to relieve menopausal symptoms.

How to Prepare: Black cohosh is typically consumed as a powdered root, herbal tea, tincture, or in supplement form (such as capsules or tablets). To make tea, dried black cohosh root is steeped in hot water for several minutes before being strained and consumed.

Dosage: The appropriate dosage of black cohosh can vary depending on factors such as age, health status, and the specific preparation being used. It's important to follow the recommended dosage on the product label or consult with a qualified herbalist or healthcare professional for personalized guidance.

How to Use: Black cohosh powder, tea, tincture, or supplements are typically taken orally. It's often used by women to support hormonal balance, relieve menopausal symptoms such as hot flashes and night sweats, and promote overall well-being.

Side Effects: Black cohosh is generally considered safe for most people when used in moderate amounts. However, some individuals may experience mild side effects such as gastrointestinal upset or allergic reactions. It may also interact with certain medications or have adverse effects in individuals with certain health conditions, such as liver disease or hormone-sensitive conditions. Pregnant or breastfeeding individuals should consult with a healthcare professional before using black cohosh supplements. It's important to use black cohosh under the guidance of a healthcare professional and to discontinue use if any adverse effects occur.

Blessed Thistle:

Definition: Blessed thistle, scientifically known as Cnicusbenedictus, is an annual or biennial herb native to the Mediterranean region but also found in other parts of Europe, Asia, and North Africa. It has been used historically in traditional medicine for its potential health benefits, particularly for digestive and liver health.

Ingredients: Blessed thistle contains various bioactive compounds, including sesquiterpene lactones (such as cnicin), flavonoids, tannins, and essential oils. These compounds are believed to contribute to the herb's medicinal properties, including its potential as a digestive tonic, appetite stimulant, and liver tonic.

How to Prepare: Blessed thistle is typically consumed as an herbal tea, tincture, or in supplement form (such as capsules or tablets). To make tea, dried blessed thistle leaves and flowers are steeped in hot water for several minutes before being strained and consumed.

Dosage: The appropriate dosage of blessed thistle can vary depending on factors such as age, health status, and the specific preparation being used. It's important to follow the recommended dosage on the product label or consult with a qualified herbalist or healthcare professional for personalized guidance.

How to Use: Blessed thistle tea, tincture, or supplements are typically taken orally. It's often used to support digestion, stimulate appetite, and promote liver health.

Side Effects: Blessed thistle is generally considered safe for most people when used in moderate amounts. However, some individuals may experience mild side effects such as gastrointestinal upset or allergic reactions. It may also interact with certain medications or have adverse effects in individuals with certain health conditions, such as hormone-sensitive conditions or bleeding disorders. Pregnant or breastfeeding individuals should consult with a healthcare professional before using blessed thistle supplements. It's important to use blessed thistle under the guidance of a healthcare professional and to discontinue use if any adverse effects occur.

THE END

www.ingramcontent.com/pod-product-compliance
Lightning Source LLC
Chambersburg PA
CBHW081559250726
48653CB00009B/3501